STEM CELL THERAPY

Before You Medicate or Operate,
Regenerate!

Drs. Paul and Patrick Baker
with Testimonials from Patients

Drs. Paul and Patrick Baker
with Testimonials from Patients

Printed in the United States of America

First Printing 2018

For permission to reproduce or to order additional copies of this book, contact Dr. Paul Baker and Dr. Patrick Baker by calling (513) 603-9969

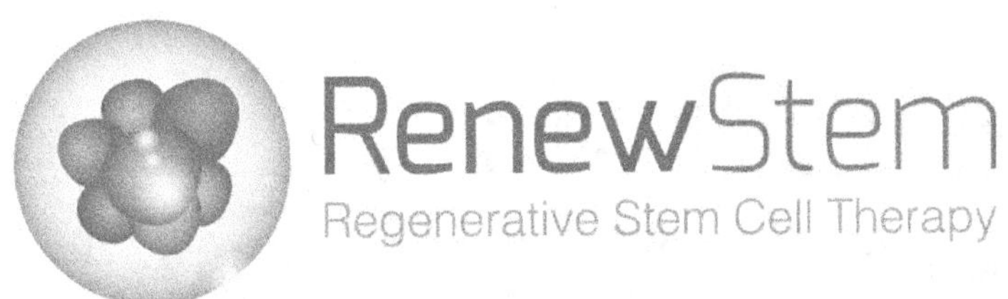

RenewStem.com

Table of Contents

Introduction

Read about the Real-Life Miraculous Effects of Stem Cells in the Face of Agonizing Pain

Science, when stated as raw facts and figures, can be quite difficult to cope with. The purpose of this book is to make you familiar with the wonders of regenerative medicine, and how it has changed lives – not those of laboratory subjects, but of actual people.

Stem Cells are here, period. And they have brought with them nothing short of miracles. The ability to restore perfect function of a body part, as if it were brand-new is truly remarkable and something to look forward to.

It doesn't matter how scarred the tissue, how damaged the joint, or how severe the trauma, Stem Cells possess a cure, and can bring your body back to the way it should be!

1

Stem Cells – Truly Regenerative Medicine

The term "Stem Cells" is often received by patients and the public with awe and amazement. It's considered too "hush-hush" to understand. The truth however, is nowhere near this.

Stem Cell research has the potential to revolutionize the way we treat many conditions, including degenerative diseases for which few effective treatments currently exist. Great hope is invested in this field by researchers, governments, and the public alike. The field has attracted priority status in many countries and has advanced rapidly. Research continues to show more and more benefits and uses of stem cell treatments.

In all simplicity, stem cells go to wherever your body needs them, and transform into whatever your body needs them for.

Stem Cells, whether they occur in the body or in the lab, are defined by two major yet simple properties:

1. They can self-renew, meaning they can generate copies of themselves upon division.
2. They can differentiate, meaning they can produce specialized cell types for specific functions in the body's organs.

The promise of stem cells as new tools for benefiting human health resides in these twin properties. Stem cells can replicate or regenerate every 28 hours for approximately 65 generations during the first 90 days!

2

Use of Stem Cell Therapies

People are quite skeptical of Stem Cell Therapy, as it is a relatively new and often misunderstood form of medicine. Nonetheless, people turn to Stem Cells out of desperation and often as a last resort. Though many people are apprehensive, due to not knowing a lot about the treatment, once they undergo it, for themselves, they often find a relief that is non-existent in other forms of treatment.

In theory, there's no limit to the types of diseases that could be treated with stem cell research. Some of these major diseases include:

1. Parkinson's Disease
2. Alzheimer's Disease
3. Type-2 Diabetes
4. Kidney Disease
5. Rheumatoid Arthritis
6. Cardiovascular Diseases
7. Spinal Cord Injuries
8. Osteoarthritis
9. Sport injuries & rotator cuff tears
10. Osteoporosis

3

Types of Stem Cell Therapies

Beyond their primary property of regeneration, Stem Cell Therapies can be split into four major types.

1. Fetal/Embryonic Stem Cell Therapies
2. Amniotic Fluid Stem Cell Therapies
3. Autologous/ Your Own Stem Cell Therapies
4. HUCT (Human Umbilical Cord Therapy)

We'll take a closer look at each of these types in the chapters that follow.

4
Fetal/Embryonic Stem Cells

Embryonic stem cells are derived from early-stage human embryos. These stem cells possess two major qualities that make them quite well suited for cellular therapy.

First, as these stem cells are obtained from early blastocysts (3-5-day-old embryo), they are at a very early developmental stage, making them highly flexible. They can become one of the more than 200 cell types that make up the human body! Given the right combination of signals, embryonic stem cells can develop into mature cells that can function as neurons, muscles, bone, blood or other needed cell types. Stem cells with such flexibility are described as "pluripotent," to indicate their high potential to differentiate into a wide variety of cell types.

Secondly, embryonic stem cells can remain within an undifferentiated state for an unlimited amount of time. This essentially gives them the property of self-renewal, allowing them to regenerate into unlimited numbers.

Much work needs to be carried out on them, both research-wise as well as legally. The extraction & use of these stem cells is an extremely controversial topic around the world, as it is seen by many as taking life from one to give to another. It is therefore the subject of several moral limitations, and illegal in the US.

RenewStem does not use the fetal/embryonic stem cell procedure due to moral and ethical issues. RenewStem is a Christian based company and would never employ using these types of immoral procedures.

5

Amniotic Fluid Stem Cells

Amniotic fluid is what surrounds a baby in the mother's womb. This fluid is highly concentrated in a number of essentials; including proteins, cytokines, and most importantly stem cells. While this fluid is mostly discharged as the "water breaks," consenting mothers of caesarian section babies can donate this fluid.

While the safe extraction of this fluid opens a lot of optimistic avenues for stem cell therapy, there are many other factors that must be considered.

Amniotic Fluid contains an unknown cell count number, and is quite difficult to extract the Stem Cells out of a large proportion of cellular debris. This makes the treatment more difficult.

6

Autologous Stem Cells

Autologous stem cells are collected from one's own body, through surgery. They may be extracted either from the bone marrow or the blood.

Extraction from Bone Marrow

A bone marrow harvest, as you may imagine, can only be performed through surgery. It occurs in an operating room and is a painful process. A surgeon inserts a large needle directly into the bone marrow cavity of bones in the lower back. Typical bone marrow harvest takes about two hours and involves the removal of one liter of bone marrow containing the stem cells. The major side effect of this procedure is discomfort at the site of the bone marrow harvest, while infrequent complications include bleeding, infection and nerve damage.

Extraction from Blood

Stem cells normally circulate in the blood in very small quantities and can be collected.

Stem cells are collected with an apheresis machine from the blood flowing through a catheter, which is inserted into a vein. Blood flows from a vein through the catheter into the apheresis machine, which separates the stem cells from the rest of the blood and then returns the blood to the patient's body. Apheresis is performed for several days until enough stem cells have been collected.

7

Human Umbilical Cord Therapy (HUCT) Stem Cells - Diving Deeper

The human umbilical cord contains several anatomical regions such as an umbilical vein, two umbilical arteries, cord lining, and Wharton's jelly, which have all been identified as giving rise to a great number of fibroblastic mesenchymal stem cells, otherwise known as Human Umbilical Cord Tissue (HUCT).

The human umbilical cord is a promising source of mesenchymal stem cells (HUCT-MSCs). Unlike bone marrow stem cells, HUCT-MSCs have a painless collection procedure as they are derived from the umbilical cord of a baby, which is otherwise discarded.

Mesenchymal stem cells (MSCs) are defined as undifferentiated cells that are capable of self-renewal and differentiation into various cell types. MSC can be isolated from bone marrow, umbilical cord blood, adipose tissue, placenta, etc. Although bone marrow has been regarded as a major source of MSC, umbilical cord blood has recently been regarded as an alternative source for isolation of MSC.

In the last 10 years, umbilical cord stem cell therapy has shown its therapeutic edge by rescuing patients with bone marrow-related deficiencies, or other errors of metabolism. Umbilical cord blood has many advantages over bone marrow because the former has a lower chance of causing a graft vs. host disease. Moreover, bone marrow stem cells are known to show changes with increasing patient age, e.g. reduction in cell count. HUCT stem cells, on the other hand, do not possess any such issues, and in fact, hold greater effectiveness against the possibility to stir up an anti-inflammatory response. This last bit is something you'll see for yourself, in the upcoming testimonials.

Finally, umbilical cord stem cells can be banked, and are thus readily available, "off the shelf", making them a convenient alternative to bone marrow sourced cells in emergency situations.

8

Musculoskeletal Issues

Musculoskeletal injuries are common in people, particularly in athletes. Even though the muscle has good regenerative ability, the extent of muscle injury can prevent complete regeneration, especially in terms of functional recovery. Severe injuries, like those originated by trauma, development of fibrous scar tissue and irreversible muscular atrophy, are examples of those situations where regeneration is limited.

People with musculoskeletal injuries may sometimes feel acute pain in their entire bodies and muscles may twitch or burn. Swelling, numbness, and tingling may be the part of the symptoms.

Common areas that are affected by musculoskeletal disorders include:

- Shoulders
- Wrists
- Hips
- Back
- Knees
- Legs

There are multiple causes for such injuries such as poor posture, accidents, repetitive motions and exertion of abundant force, etc. but at the end of the day they lead to serious, life-altering problems such as:

- Tendinitis

- Carpal tunnel syndrome

- Osteoarthritis

- Rheumatoid arthritis

- Fibromyalgia

- Bone fractures

- Muscle / Tendon strain

In such cases – even if you're not put off by the idea of your bones being drilled into – extraction of stem cells from within your own self is of little use, since the body has already exhausted its resources; therefore, one must turn towards HUCT stem cells.

9

Benefits of HUCT Stem Cells

Here's a list of the many benefits HUCT Stem Cells can provide:

- Umbilical cord tissue provides an abundant supply of mesenchymal stem cells.

- Since HUCT mesenchymal stem cells are immune system privileged, cell rejection is not an issue.

- HUCT stem cells have the best anti-inflammatory activity, immune modulating capacity, and ability to stimulate regeneration.

- HUCT stem cells can be administered multiple times over the course of months in uniform dosages that contain high cell counts.

- There is a growing body of evidence showing that umbilical cord-derived mesenchymal stem cells are more robust than mesenchymal stem cells from other sources.

10

Patient Testimonials

All the information that we have shared in the previous chapters has been our best effort to educate you on the research and benefits of Stem Cell Therapy. We'd love to share some of our success stories from patients who have undergone the treatment. Please read their stories, take in their experiences and reach out to us with any questions you may have.

Conchi's Story

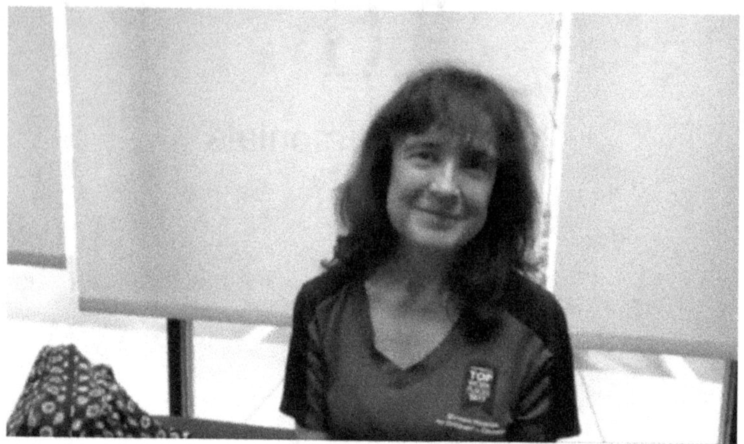

Conchi, a nurse at Shriner's Hospital for Children, had stem cell injections after suffering from severe shoulder and hip pain.

After I had the injections of stem cells, the pain went away. So right now, I can say that I'm a hundred percent pain-free. It's been three weeks now.

I was skeptical, but I trusted Dr. Baker, and I thought I would give it a try instead of taking pills all the time. Now, I can work my shifts!

Barbara's Story

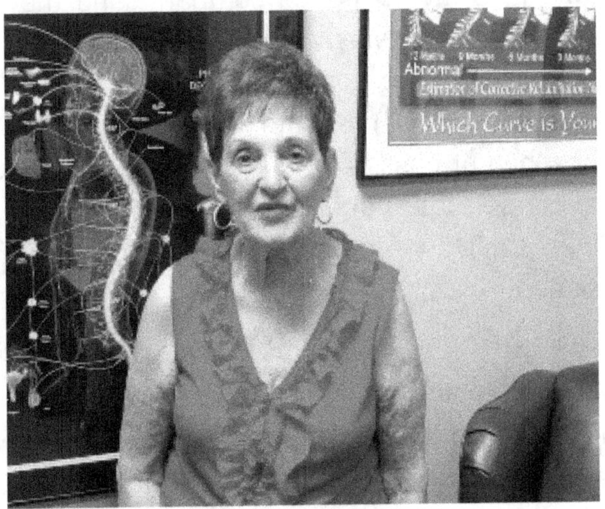

After a very athletic youth, Barbara began suffering from right knee pain more than 15 years ago. A failed series of "gel" injections over several years led her to investigate and receive Stem Cell Therapy.

About 15 years ago, I had an injection in my right knee, and it really helped me – for a year. When it wore off, my knee was bone on bone. It got worse. I know a lot of people my age who had knee replacement, but I didn't do that because I knew I was going to suffer with it.

I had a really bad experience, almost 2 years ago. I was telling my doctor at Christ Hospital about my knee and told him that I wasn't having a knee replacement. So, he sent me to an orthopedic doctor at Christ Hospital who recommended a "gel" injection.

We had to take it to my insurance company, and they decided, instead of me having one injection, I had to have three. I had one injection three weeks in a row, each one costing $1,200. The shots hurt so bad that I came within an inch of passing out, and my face turned white. The doctor sent the nurse to get the oxygen. But after all of that, I might've taken just a drink of water. Nothing happened!

That's when Dr. Patrick started telling me about stem cells, and I called my son, an anesthesiologist, right away. I was very apprehensive. Doctor Jeremy is very meticulous. They conducted an ultrasound of my knee, because it was bone on bone. There wasn't much in there to work with. He used the ultrasound, looking for a soft place to get it through my knee.

I knew the test for the procedure would be if I could make it to bed after having the Stem Cell Therapy. All my bedrooms are upstairs in my house. So, for two stairs, I come down the stairs one foot at a time every morning. And I go up at night, with my hands on the step, getting up.

My Stem Cell Therapy was done on a Saturday. Then on Sunday night when I had to go to bed, I wondered whether something had happened. I could finally go up the steps!

Rebecca's Story

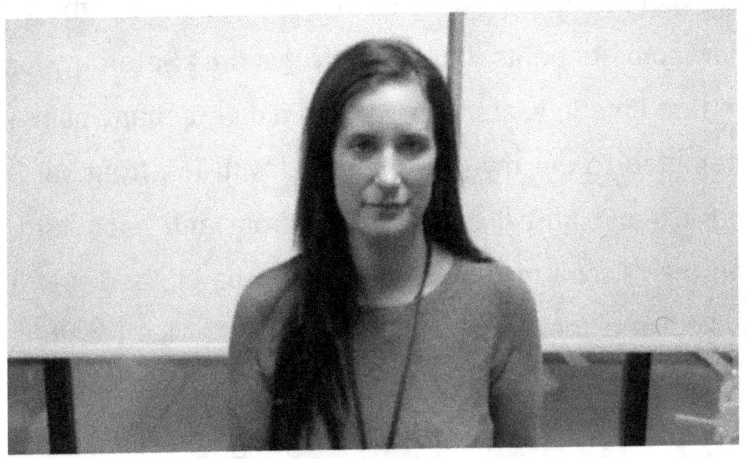

Rebecca suffered from a severe case of illiopsoas bursitis for more than five years.

After doing a lot of heavy lifting over the years, I had a lot of pain in my left back, and I couldn't figure out where it was coming from. We did figure out it was coming from my psoas, and it pretty much restricted everything I did, especially going up and down steps, or anything that required me to lift my leg, e.g. walking a lot, pushing anything like a lawn mower, etc.

On average, my pain level was at a 6, but if I did something like go upstairs, it would increase to 8 or 9.

I had my Stem Cell injections 10 days ago. I thought stem cells would take at least a couple of months to show some benefits, but honestly this past Saturday, for the first time in years, I got up and didn't feel any pain. I attempted to cut my grass, starting with the front yard, and it didn't hurt. I cut my entire front and back yard, and then I took my son to a pumpkin patch, and then I walked at a festival downtown for hours. I kept waiting for the pain, and it never came, it was very strange so I'm excited to see where this is going. It still has not been sore. I didn't even ice afterward, which normally I do after doing anything. I'm seeing benefits already!

Sue's Story

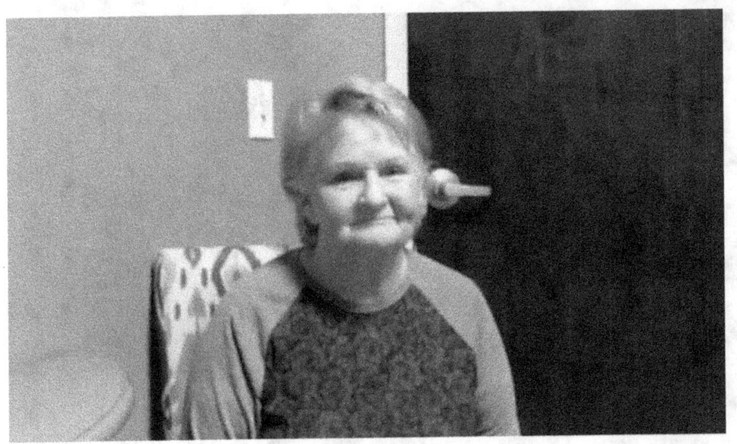

After suffering from knee pain for quite some time, Sue turned to Stem Cell Therapy for relief.

Before my injection, my pain level was at a 10. I could hardly go up and down the steps. It was like one step a time, and it would still hurt quite a bit. But now my knee is more fluid, and I can go up and down the steps quite well now. It feels much better. I'm looking forward to more energy and also fluidness in the knee. My yoga is much better and my pain is around 2 or minus 2!

Dr. Paul told me that I'm going to continue to improve because the stem cells reach a maximum peak of healing in 90 days.

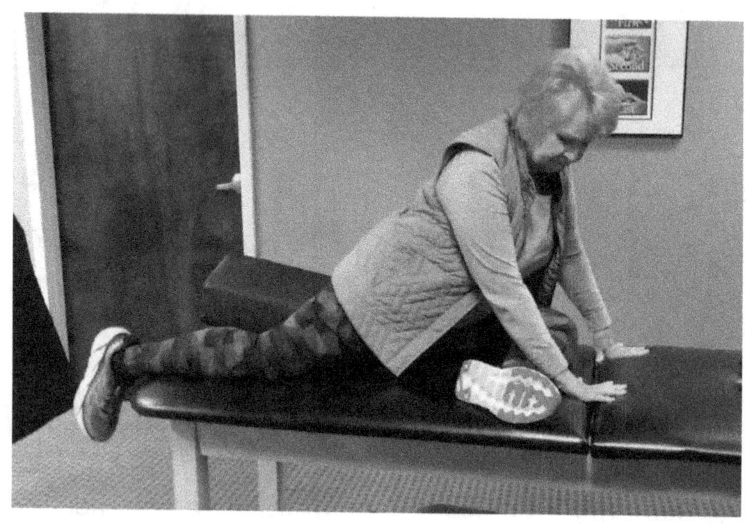

I do a lot of yoga, and this is called a pigeon pose.

Before I had the injection, I couldn't do this. Now, I can lie this way, and it's still not perfect, but it's getting there.

Wayne's Story

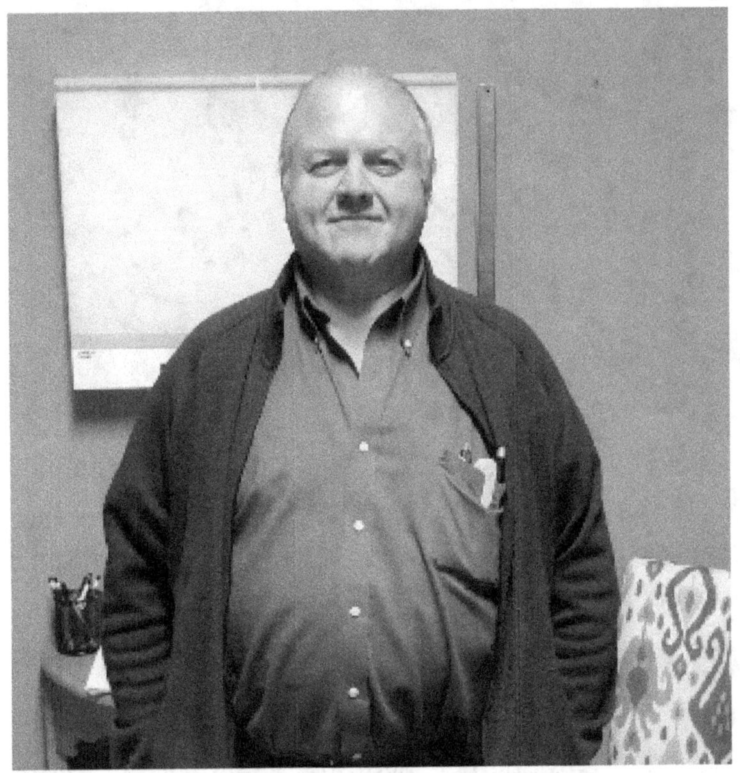

Wayne suffered from shoulder pain and had Stem Cell injections two months ago.

I feel fantastic! No pain, no aches, everything's working good. Prior to my injection, on a scale of 1-10, my pain level was a 12. Today? Zero!

Mark's Story

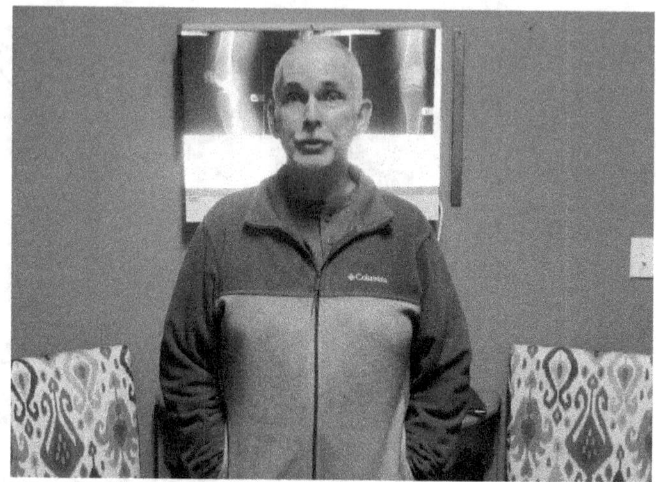

Mark had undergone a different, much more invasive, Stem Cell procedure a couple of years ago for his hip, and recently underwent injections with the Bakers.

I got stem cells put in both my hips and both my knees. I was a little anxious because I had stem cells put in my left hip by a different procedure a couple of years ago.

The old way to do this was invasive, meaning a little bit scary. They had to drill on six sides in my pelvis to harvest my stem cells out my bone marrow. You're awake during this – so it's invasive!

I had four umbilical cord stem-cells injections done by Dr. Jeremy. I did not have to go to a hospital or a big clinic. Dr. Jeremy was just wonderful.

I was very anxious coming in after what I went through a couple of years ago. I had four needles, so I was worried. But the pain was very minimal, just a pin prick.

Now, I'm standing up and talking after the procedure, feeling the same way as I was when I walked through the door!

Patt's Story

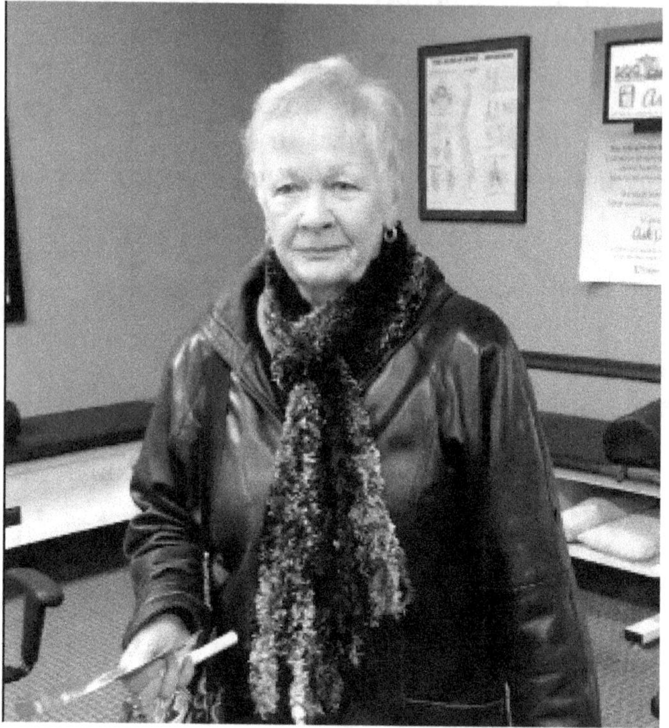

Patt has been a chronic back pain sufferer.

I walked out to my car and, when I walked in here, I had pain in my back, and when I walked out, the pain was gone!

Barb's Story

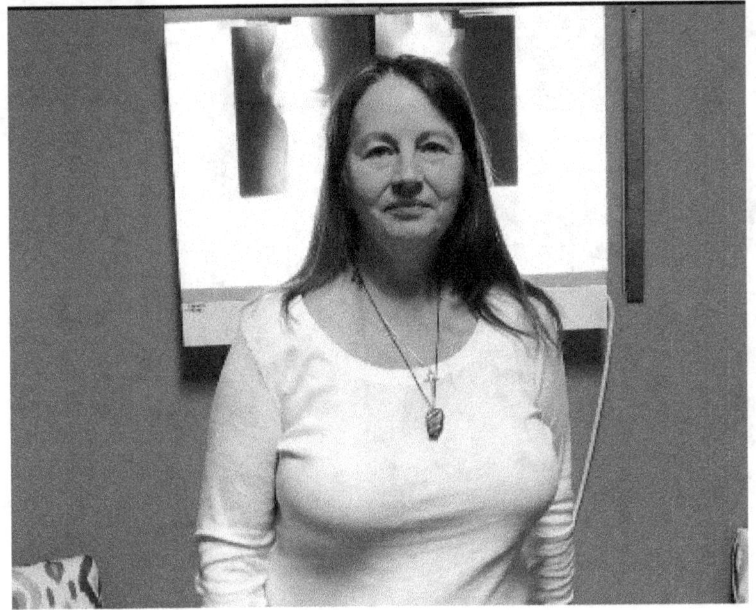

Barb suffered from hip pain for quite some time.

I just had both of my hips injected with Stem Cells. It was really simple, almost like a piece of cake! It just a little prick, you numb the area, take a little of my blood, mix it. One side was a little pricklier than the other, but otherwise it was fine.

I was nervous coming here, not knowing what to expect, but it was a piece of cake.

Ken's Story

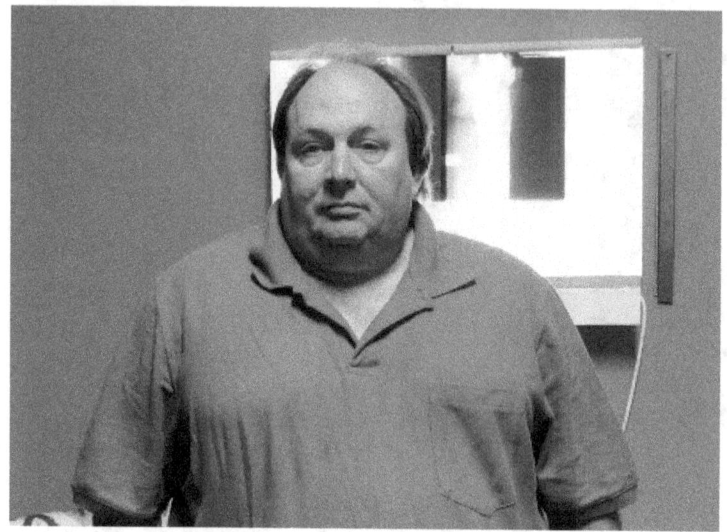

Ken just had an injection of stem cells into his hip.

It was quite painless, just a numbed area with a needle on it. Dr. Baker told me that the neat thing about my procedure was that it was ultrasound guided, so we could actually see the fluid go right into the joint space. That technique is used because it gets the stem cells & PRP right in the exact position where we need it.

Right now, I feel a little better. So far so good!

Gene's Story

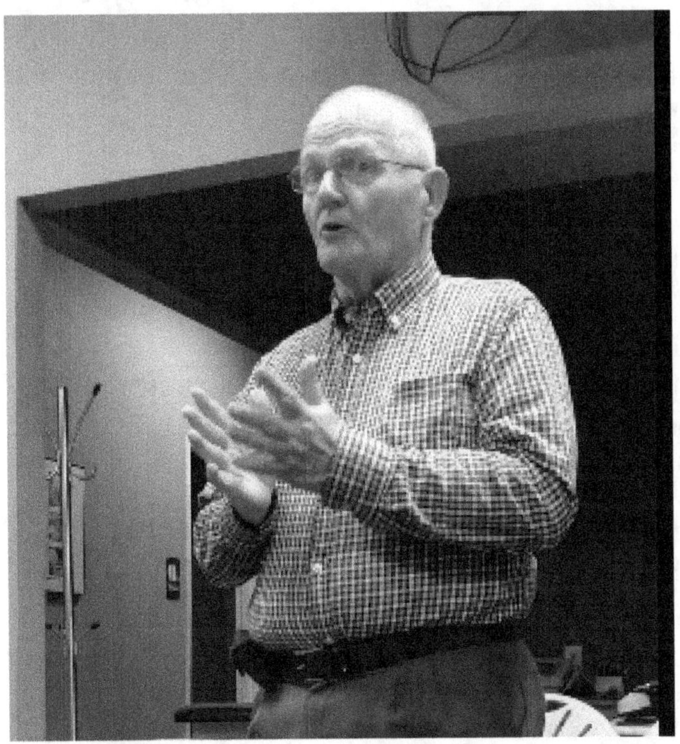

Gene had injections in his left knee after years of pain, a near-death experience following orthoscopic surgery and a knee replacement – none of which improved his pain.

It started in 2005, when I lived in Tennessee and we were cutting down a tree for a friend — we cut it up and sold fireplace lengths. I picked up a piece that had drove down the hill, and was bringing it back up. I caught my foot in a vine, and rather than throw the piece, I maintained my balance.

I heard something that sounded like a gun going off, but it was my left knee. I had torn cartilage. I had pain immediately and went to the doctor. They tried all kinds of wraps and anything that my insurance company would pay for. Nothing seemed to help.

So, about a year after that, I was told I needed to go to Knoxville Sports Orthopedics to have them take care of it. And they did an orthoscopic surgery on my knee. After that, my doctor said I would have pain for a few days. I then had to go to therapy. And after my third trip, they told me there wouldn't be any therapy that day.

After driving 35 miles to get there, I was told I may have some blood clot problems. My wife called my lung doctor and asked for any tests that could rule out blood clots. I was told if I could make it to the hospital in the next hour, some tests could be done on us.

I went to the hospital, walked in and walked up two flights of stairs. When I got up there, I was told to wait. They called me, and I walked back with a nurse. When they performed the test, they told me to sit still because I had blood clots in my lungs. The lung doctor said, he wasn't sure if I would live for more than 2 days.

But I overcame that and went back to see the Orthopedic doctor. I thought he was going to cry, he looked as if he was ready to shed tears. I had to comfort him! He said he wouldn't do any more things on me, because he couldn't stand to lose a patient. What he had done was that he punctured holes in my bone so that stem cells would come out and regenerate the area. It didn't work.

Anyway, a year later, I had to go to Ohio, where I had a knee replacement. They said it would take care of the pain. This was in 2007. Until about 2 months ago, I had the same pain that I had originally.

In April, I asked the doctor as to why I still had pain after knee replacement. I showed him the knee, and he told me that it wasn't a knee – it was a tendon. So, by then, I had spent on $30,000 on a knee replacement, and other things, and it was of no good.

I had heard about stem cells in Tennessee. A friend of mine had stem cells therapy, but it was a kind in which they take the fat out of the body. She said it's very painful, but she also said that it helped. So, I started saving my money once again.

We heard about it here and saw the benefits of younger stem cells. I'm 75 years old so I'm just about the bottom of the chart! And I thought that young stem cells might be the answer.

On September 30, I had stem cells injected. Two days later I told my wife, "That pain is gone!" Up until that time, if I was down the basement, I had to step down one foot at a time.

On Sunday, our son was at our house, and my wife told him to go down to the basement! I said to him, let me show you how things used to be. I started running down the steps. My son couldn't believe it, and he came down the way I used to – one step at a time. Fifty-two years old, and his knees were in worse shape than mine.

We had a friend, two doors down, who had siding damage on his house. My wife and I used to do siding work, and I told him that I would like to replace that. He told me to give it a go. To match the siding, I had to climb up the ladder. And when the guy took off running up steps, I just took off after him. I got up 15 steps and realized that I hadn't even touched the handrail.

I would very much recommend stem cells.

I've had surgeries so many times. When I had the knee replacement, and for two days I couldn't get out of bed, because what they gave me to put me out. But then they transferred me to a nursing home where I spent 30 days, getting therapy on my knees. I know that the therapist there followed the motto, "no pain, no gain", and I had a lot of gain! But I highly recommend stem cell therapy.

Steve's Story

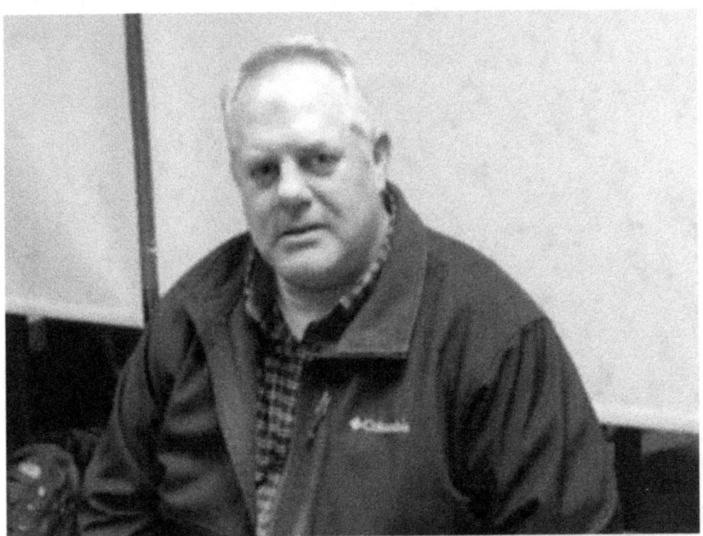

Steve had his left knee injected three months ago. Before he received his treatment, his pain level was at an 8 and walking caused a lot of grinding and pain.

Now I'm not having pain. In fact, on the day of injection, I went to an auction site, walked some rough ground. It was perfectly fine. During the injection I felt a little pressure. That night when I went up my stairs, that knee didn't grind for the first time, in I don't know how long!

Looking at the X-ray of my knee, there's a bigger gap there. I can see it, but more importantly I can feel it.

[The procedure] had a profound effect on me. I went to Church after that, and felt God gave me a second chance.

Paul's Story

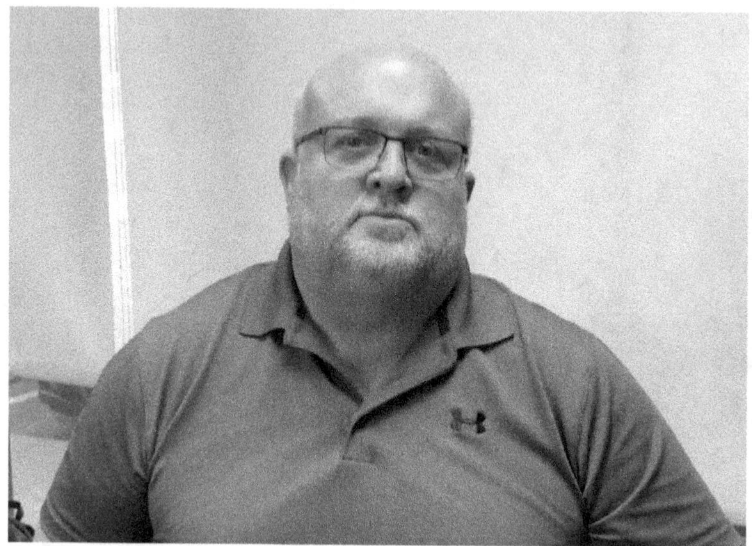

Paul had his low back, right hip and right knee injected. His right hip had very severe degenerative changes and only a 20% chance for success for treatment.

Before my treatment, I had to take a lot of anti-inflammatories. It was painful. I didn't know if I could do this. I had sharp pain in my hip, and in my knee. I didn't want to move. I tried to stay still.

Pre-injection, if I had to go to the kitchen or to the bathroom, I made it worth my while because I wasn't going back again.

The injection was really very simple. It was like a flu shot. I was very comfortable. There wasn't any pain, but the original pain was there. I had my injection on a Friday, but on the next Wednesday I realized there was no pain most of the day. Since the following Thursday, there hasn't been any pain.

My mobility has changed quite a bit. I have even video-taped myself daily. After Thursday, it has always been good. I used to walk, one step at a time, up the stairs.

Now, I don't think twice about going to the car. Back in the gym, they wanted me to do cardio because I didn't want to move my hip or knee. Now, I'm trying to find a larger range (of exercises).

Pre-injection, my pain was over nine, if not ten. Especially the hip – the hip was always the harder pain. The knee was underneath it.

Post injection, three months today, my pain is at a zero or one! One is probably my age and weight pain.

I have already recommended this treatment to family and friends. I don't know how many people on Facebook have asked me and followed-up with me about it.

I had three other doctors telling me, "You're not a candidate." And here I am: I'm not in pain now at all.

Deborah's Story

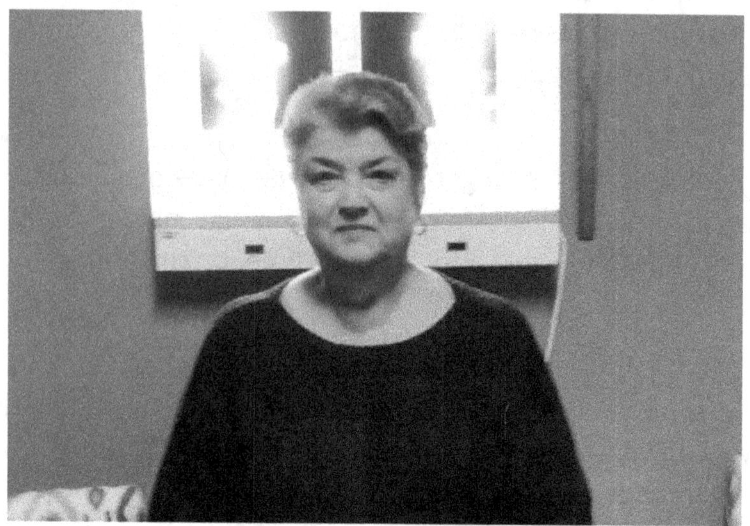

Deborah had her stem cell injections in her right knee.

I can't believe the difference. It's amazing. Oh, my goodness, it was bad before. Pain-wise, it was over a 10. But, now, it's been about five weeks since my injection, and I can go up and down stairs without even thinking about it. I don't have to take one step at a time anymore!

I still have a little bit more to go, but I'm thrilled with how this went through me.

I would absolutely recommend the treatment. It's just amazing. The first week, I really didn't see a difference. If you just give it some time, it's going to work for you.

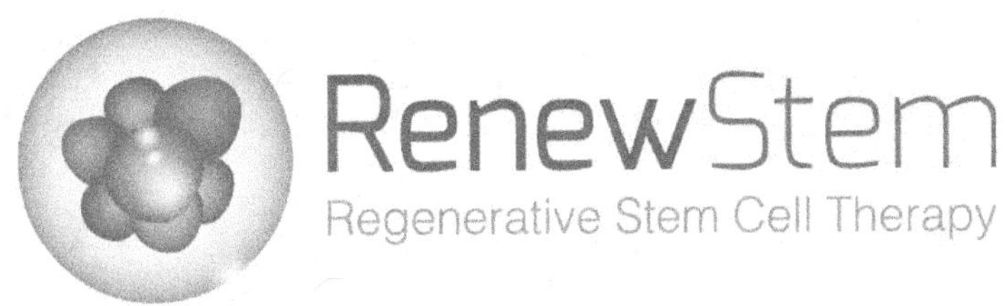

For more information about stem cell therapy, please contact Dr. Paul Baker and Dr. Patrick Baker by calling (513) 603-9969 or visit renewstem.com.